PUSH-UP PROGRESSION WORKOUT FOR A STRONGER CORE

PUSH-UP PROGRESSION WORKOUT FOR A STRONGER CORE

A Twelve Push-up Journey

Shaun Zetlin

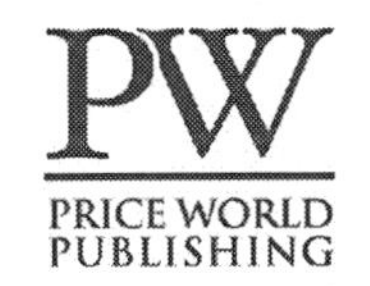

Prior to beginning any exercise program, you must consult with your physician. You must also consult your physician before increasing the intensity of your training. The information in this book is intended for healthy individuals. Any application of the recommended material in this book is at the sole risk of the reader, and at the reader's discretion. Responsibility of any injuries or other adverse effects resulting from the application of any of the information provided within this book is expressly disclaimed.

Price World Publishing
1300 W Belmont Ave Ste 20G
Chicago, IL 60657-3200
www.PriceWorldPublishing.com

Photos by: Rebecca Weiss Photography http://www.rebeccaweiss.com/

ISBN: 9781619841840

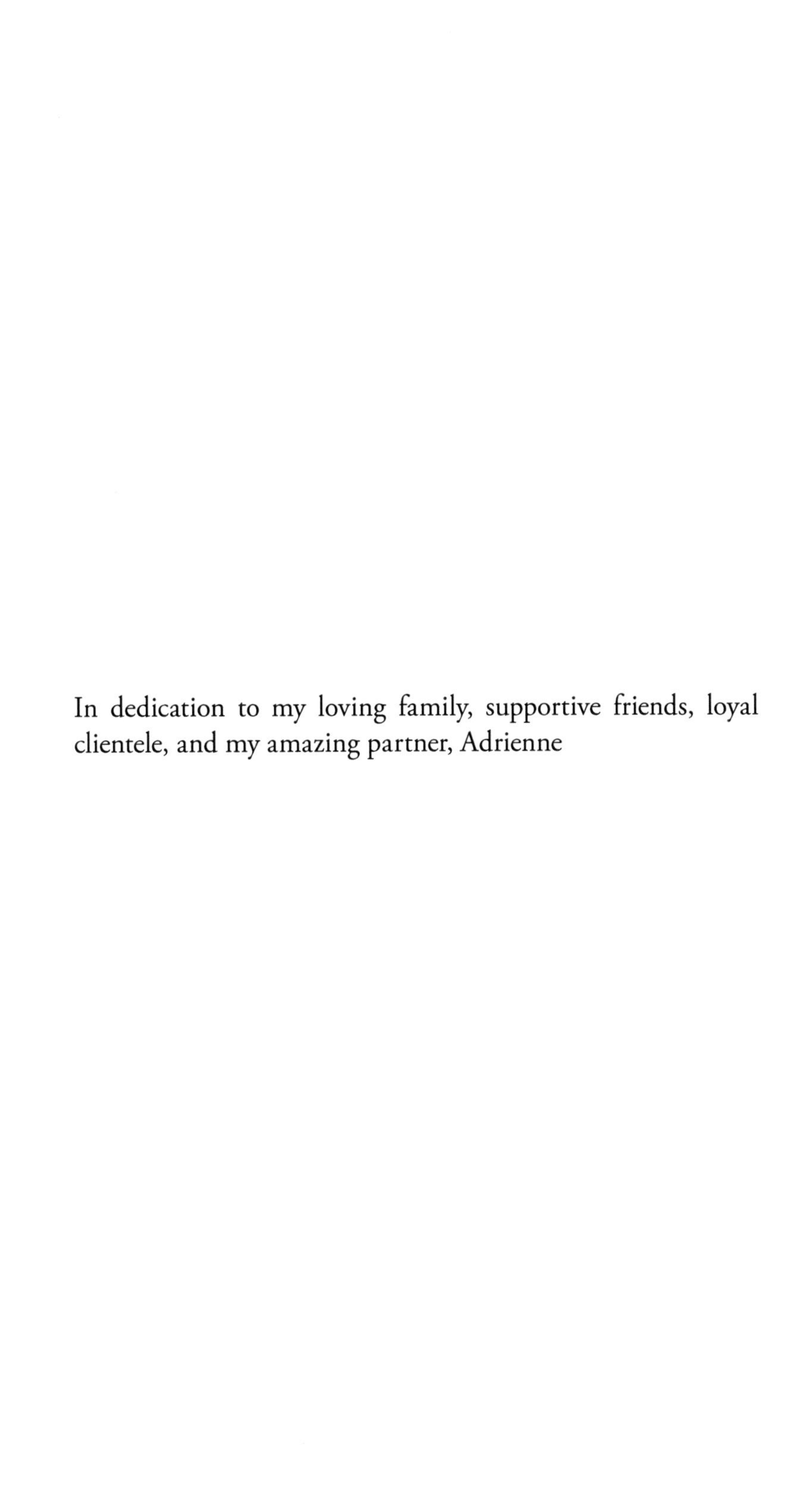

In dedication to my loving family, supportive friends, loyal clientele, and my amazing partner, Adrienne

Table of Contents

Introduction

"Push-up Progression Workout for a Stronger Core" speaks to the benefits of progression while executing the otherwise "traditional push-up" by performing it in various ways and via multiple techniques. This book will discuss how crucial the push-up is in regards to training the core, upper body, and lower body.

Anyone and everyone should read this book because the push-up can benefit anyone who is seeking more core stabilization, better posture, more power, stronger stability in their joints, and more strength in their upper and lower body.

While you discover how to improve your push-up technique, a main goal of this book is to inspire you to appreciate the benefits of refining your push-up approach in meeting your overall fitness training goals. You will not only become more advanced at performing the push-up, but will gain increased core stabilization and functionally improved posture.

Mastering the push-up is important because while some individuals can press heavy weights at the gym, their actual strength may not compare when it comes to performing the push-up. Similarly, both the beginner and professional alike may be unaware of the expansive value the push-up provides to conditioning the entire body.

Beyond the common desire to have stronger arms and shoulders, most individuals need to improve their core strength and posture. Unbeknownst to many, the push-up can address all of those needs. The different levels of progression of push-ups will work stability, muscle isolation, isometrics, strength, power, and function.

Surely, if one was able to do a variety of a single exercise from the comfort of their own home, while addressing the desired results mentioned above, the benefits would be plentiful. Simply put, the push-up can be an amazing alternative for those who don't regularly make it to the gym. For that reason, "Push-up Progression Workout for a Stronger Core" can benefit people with even the most hectic of lifestyles.

Core

Core is a very popular word these days in the world of fitness. Most of us have probably seen or heard this term used frequently. While most of us know that having a stronger core is fundamental, let's take a more detailed look into why a stronger core is crucial for everyone.

What is core?

Core can be best characterized as the central location of the body that consists of your entire spine (cervical, thoracic, and lumbar), the pelvic girdle and hips. Therefore, the core can be defined as your entire body except for your arms and legs.

Anatomy of the Core

The muscles of the core can be classified into distinct categories based on their function of either stabilizing or providing movement for your body.

The muscles below stabilize the core:

Transverse Abdominis
Internal Oblique
Pelvic Floor
Multifidus
Diaphragm

Transversospinalis

These muscles provide movement to the core:

Rectus Abdominis
External Oblique
Latissimus Dorsi
Erector Spinae
Iliopsoas
Hip Adductors
Hip Abductors

All of the core muscles in these two categories must work together as one functional unit to provide optimal stabilization and movement for the body. These muscles must be trained correctly for optimal functional activity or compensations most likely will occur from inefficient movements. Performing inefficient movements consistently over time will create more opportunities for the body to become injured. Therefore, it's vital to train the core muscles first for stabilization. Then, once these muscles have become stable, the next step would be to train the core muscles that provide movement. For example, when starting a core training routine, you always want to perform a plank first. The plank incorporates most of the stabilization muscles. After your core stabilization muscles are strong from doing the plank, then you could attempt some crunches. Crunches engage the core movement muscles. Therefore, the formula for a stronger core should always be training the stabilization muscles first, and the movement muscles secondarily.

The push-ups in this book include the core muscles that provide stabilization. Moreover, some of the more advanced exercises featured later in this book include a variety of the core movement muscles.

Core Function

The core can be considered to be the first muscle that becomes engaged with movement. It is the center of gravity for the body. The stabilization core muscles in your body must function with the best possible efficiency in order to operate with optimal strength, endurance, and power. If these stabilization core muscles are weak it will most likely result in injuries, namely, developing into chronic lower back pain. Therefore, individuals who do not strength-train their core stabilization muscles are more likely to increase their risk for injuries than those who don't. These stabilization muscles can be trained through utilizing the push-up exercises in this book.

The core stabilization muscles are composed of Type 1 muscle fibers. They respond best to tension engagement of the core for 10 to 20 seconds per implementation. If the core movement muscles are inadequate, then they cannot provide the proper role to aid with the core stabilization muscles. The bottom line is: *if the core stabilization and movement muscles are all working at optimal levels, not only will you have proper function in your core muscles, but overall you will have more strength, endurance, and power with all the other muscles in your body while performing any movement.* For example, if an individual is attempting a traditional push-up and has very strong core stabilization muscles, but lacks strength in their upper body, their core strength will help their upper body muscles become stronger by performing the push-up on a consistent basis. This cycle can even apply to weight training, as developing a stronger core from push-ups can assist with pressing more weight at the gym. In fact, performing the push-ups in this book will produce more overall strength and function in any exercise you perform at the gym.

Posture

Since the core can be defined as the entire spine, having optimal stabilization and movement in our core muscles is critical for the best possible posture. However, as mentioned above, when training the core for optimal posture, core stabilization muscles must be strength-trained first and core movement muscles trained secondarily.

Many of us struggle with good posture and thus engage in compensations when we exercise or perform daily life activities, which again can only result in a variety of injuries. Not to mention, bad posture is not an aesthetically pleasing look.

There are multiple activities that contribute to terrible posture. Primarily, sitting excessively in a chair, which so many professions require, wreaks havoc on one's posture. Try your best not to sit for more than one to two hours at a time. Be sure to take intermittent breaks by standing up and crossing your hands on your chest. Next, with your feet positioned at shoulder-width, perform a backbend (hyperextension), holding for 10 seconds for four repetitions. This stretch will provide some relief and help improve posture, although it won't provide optimal core stabilization strength. The push-ups listed in this book*, however, will increase strength to your core stabilization and movement muscles and help improve functionally-optimal posture. Remember to do your best to always be aware of and practice proper posture while you sit, walk, or perform any other daily activity for correct efficient movements.

*Note, if you suffer from any posture disorder please skip to the Muscular Imbalance section of this book before performing any of the push-ups listed.

Drawing-In Maneuver

When strength training the core stabilization and movement muscles it is more beneficial to "draw in" your abdominals right before performing a core exercise. To perform this correctly, "suck" in your abdominal muscles towards the spine. This maneuver can create better support for the pelvis and therefore more overall strength in your core. Moreover, drawing-in helps aid your spine in finding neutral position, a common starting point of any push-up. By maintaining a neutral spinal position during push-ups, you will develop better posture, muscle balance, and stabilization.

Push-ups

What is a Push-up?

A push-up is an anaerobic exercise that is a body-weight movement. It is performed in the prone (chest down) position with elbows bent at 90 degrees, using the arms to lower and raise your torso. The gravity and resistance that your body provides during this exercise creates functional and overall strength. Functional strength can best be defined as effectively producing stabilization and movement to the body with daily activities.

Push-ups can be considered a “moving plank” since the core is utilized for strength just as much as the upper body is during performance. Correct push-ups should be executed with the upper body, torso, and lower body moving as one unit. Push-ups are a tremendously beneficial exercise due to the multiple joint and muscle groups they recruit. Moreover and most importantly, push-ups are a true test of strength, stability, endurance, and power. *Not to mention: push-ups can be performed almost anywhere without the need of joining a gym or leaving the comfort of your own home.*

Benefits of Push-ups

Push-ups build lean muscle in your anterior, medial, and posterior deltoid muscles; pectoralis major and pectoralis minor muscles; and triceps. Additionally, other push-up variations listed in this book engage your rhomboids, the latissimus dorsi, rotator cuffs, hip flexors, erector spinae, gluteus maximus muscles, hamstrings, and calves.

While the push-up is considered one of the most popular exercises in the world, many still perform them with incorrect form and are not properly engaging the right muscles for strength, stabilization, and power. Furthermore, with so many push-up variations out there—some with supportive inanimate objects—it can prove difficult to perform the seemingly simple push-up with optimal efficiency. With proper posture, form, and core engagement, this book will show you how you can more quickly see physical results from every push-up you execute, with improved musculature in areas you may not have expected!

The push-up and the core should work together in perfect harmony for optimal performance when all of these specific muscles are appropriately engaged. They both assist in utilizing one's strengths to create the ideal exercise for so many different training techniques. For example, if you have a weak core, but a very strong upper-body pressing ability, attempting a traditional push-up might at first prove challenging when trying to engage your core. It might also be difficult to find or keep a neutral spinal position while performing the push-up. However, eventually the core stabilization muscles will become stronger and inherently, if the core is properly engaged during every push-up exercise featured in this book, so will the rest of your body!

Neutral Spinal Position

The neutral spinal position can be defined as having the top of your shoulders, mid-back, and gluteus maximus muscles perfectly aligned. This spinal position must be executed during every push-up for proper core and muscle engagement. The neutral spinal position produces efficient movements for the body and helps develop optimal posture. Finally, and most importantly, this positioning in your spine encourages more overall strength for your body when performing movement patterns.

When attempting the neutral spinal position, "draw in" your abdominals and engage your gluteus muscles. Remember to be especially cautious not to allow your lower back form an inward curve, causing your hips to drop excessively. Similarly, do not round your back, which raises your gluteus maximus muscles higher than your hips. Both of these incorrect methods can cause stress to your lower back, jeopardizing the development of functional core strength in the stabilization and movement muscles.

Tips on Finding Your Neutral Spinal Position

Mirror - The mirror can be a great tool to help find the neutral spinal position if you are unsure of how it should feel or look. It can be hard to confirm your alignment, particularly when in the prone (chest down) position. Don't be shy about checking yourself in the mirror until you are confident that you have mastered this spinal positioning throughout the exercise.

Picture - Have a friend or family member take a picture of you in the neutral spinal position. This picture can serve two purposes. First, it can aid as a useful prompt to help you remember what your body should look like in this position.

Secondly, the act of finding the correct position can actually help your muscles "remember" how to find and maintain the position better. Be sure to study the picture and refine your posture until perfect, even if multiple pictures are necessary, until you obtain that perfect shape. Remember: it is crucial that you master the neutral spinal position before starting your push-up journey.

Tips to Maximize Your Efforts

Gluteus Maximus

You may not realize it, but the gluteus maximus muscles can serve as a functional support system while performing a push-up. Additionally, actively engaging your gluteus maximus muscles helps perform the push-up more easily. It's crucial that these muscles are strong because when they are weak, various compensations can occur in the body. Compensations can lead to the over-stressing of certain muscles, which can result in strain or injury. Specifically, muscular imbalances in the pelvis can prevent you from performing and maintaining the neutral spinal position during push-ups. Stronger gluteus maximus muscles help prevent these muscular imbalances. Another benefit of engaging your gluteus maximus muscles during push-ups is that lean muscle can be created, which provides these muscles with an aesthetically pleasing look as a result.

Breathing

Taking proper breaths is essential for achieving the best possible strength and power while performing push-ups. To execute properly, take in a deep breath as you descend into a push-up. Next, rise up and breathe out solidly as you return to the starting position. You may want to take multiple breaths during the push-up if needed to accomplish more core engagement and overall strength. Don't be afraid to make your breaths audible, too, both to help you execute them more fully and to maintain consistency while executing the push-up.

Log Your Results

It can be very beneficial to keep records of your push-ups for multiple reasons. Foremost, writing down your results can help you acknowledge and remember your achievements. It's a wonderful feeling to look back and recall your push-up accomplishments and see how you have progressed. Secondly, think of how much further you can go! Keeping records of your progress (and struggles) can help you define your next goal, whether big or small, inspiring you to work out harder. Lastly, sometimes a number says it all. During your push-up routines, writing down the actual number of push-ups you have performed can serve as a gratifying and inspiring reminder. Consider using a notebook, composition book, file on your computer or PDA, or even just a piece of paper—anything that conveniently helps you track and define your results and goals and helps keep you going!

Safety Disclaimer

You know your body better than anyone. It's vital to listen to your body before, during, and after exercising. Please do not hesitate to consult your Sports Medicine Physician if you feel any kind of pain when performing the exercises in this book. Pain is never a good thing while exercising and it's your body's method of letting you know that something could be wrong. If you have a history of high blood pressure, hypertension, heart disease, or any other chronic disease, please consult your physician before exercising to confirm that you are healthy enough to perform this program. Additionally, if you experience any sharp or intense pain in your shoulders, lower back, wrists, or anywhere else while attempting these push-ups, please stop and contact your physician.

Before You Begin

I'd like to take you on a push-up journey. A journey in conquering twelve different types of push-ups for stronger core stabilization and movement muscles, and developing more lean muscle in your upper and lower body. This journey will also promote more overall strength and better posture, and will provide better function to your muscles. Much like life, this is a journey and not a destination. There is absolutely no timetable or urgency to complete the twelve push-ups immediately. There are no inanimate objects needed such as chair or stability ball. The only tools necessary on your push-up journey are: your own body weight, passionate desire, and consistent patience. Remember that exercising is as much mental as it is physical. For that reason, before attempting any push-up on your journey, say these words to yourself repeatedly and commit them to your memory: "I know I can do this." Instead of only passively thinking you are able to perform these push-ups, know in your soul that you can. Believe in the benefits they'll yield. Embrace the challenge for the gratification that exists on the other side. Now here we go!

"The Focused Five"

Before taking the starting position of any of the push-ups below, get into the habit of remembering and applying these five points of focus. Consider them your mantras, and let them always be your sidekick:

- Maintain a neutral spinal position
- Do not lean or hike your hips upwards
- Engage your gluteus maximus
- "Draw in" your abdominals

- Utilize your downward inhaling / upward exhaling breath

Even though these points are not listed with every exercise below, remember to apply them at all times! They are the baseline starting blocks to your Twelve Push-up Journey.

The Twelve Push-ups Journey

1. Isometric Hold Push-ups

This push-up is an excellent isometric movement for strengthening your core stabilization muscles and gluteus maximus muscles. These isometric holds will also create lean muscle in your upper body and assist in developing stronger tendons to aide your rotator cuff. Moreover, this exercise will help you progress to performing all the other push-ups listed.

Starting Position: Begin by getting down on the floor with your chest facing the ground and your knees, feet, and legs together and your heels up. Your hands should be positioned slightly more than shoulder-width apart and your elbows only slightly bent.

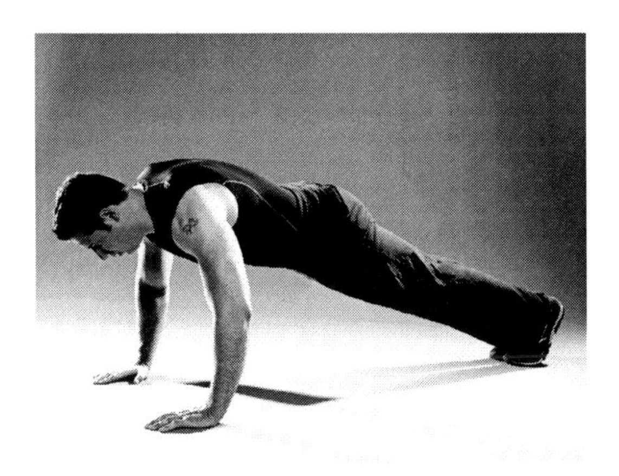

To Perform: Hold this position while slightly bending the elbows and with the knees, feet, and legs together. Your heels should be off the ground and rotated slightly forward. There is no need to lower your upper body to the ground since the main goal in this exercise is to achieve more core and upper body stability.

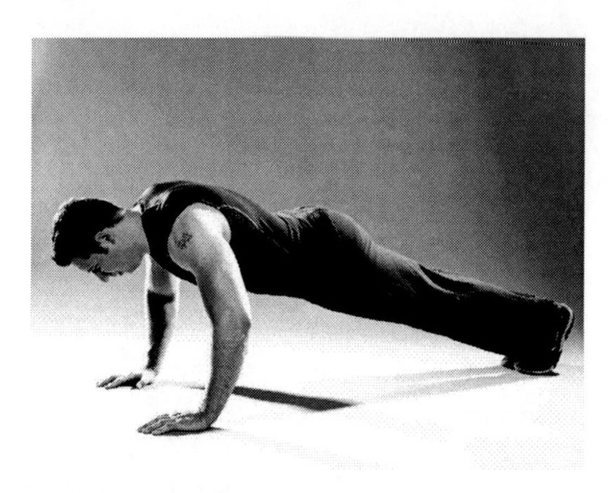

Beginner: Three sets, 10 seconds each
Intermediate: Four sets, 30 seconds each
Advanced: Five sets, 60 seconds each

Rest time between sets should be 10 to 30 seconds for recovery.

Tips: If holding this stance is too difficult, situate your hands wider to make it easier for your body to stabilize the hold. Additionally, the wider you keep your hands apart, the more you will incorporate your shoulders to create that "broader" look. Apply The Focused Five.

2. Traditional Push-ups

After successfully mastering the Isometric Hold Push-up position, it's time to attempt the ever-popular Military Push-up. Before even attempting this push-up, do not be consumed with how far you are able to lower your body. Range of motion and overall strength will come. For now, focus on your breath (as noted in "Tips"), engage your abdominal and gluteus maximus muscles, and embrace the challenge your own body weight provides. It's best to remember that you are pushing your own body weight. Along with the general benefits, this exercise specifically builds lean muscle in these primary movers: the anterior and medial deltoid muscles, pectoralis major and pectoralis minor muscles, triceps, and gluteus maximus.

Starting Position: Position yourself with your chest facing the ground and your hands a little more than shoulder-width apart. Your knees, feet, and legs should be together to promote optimal core stability.

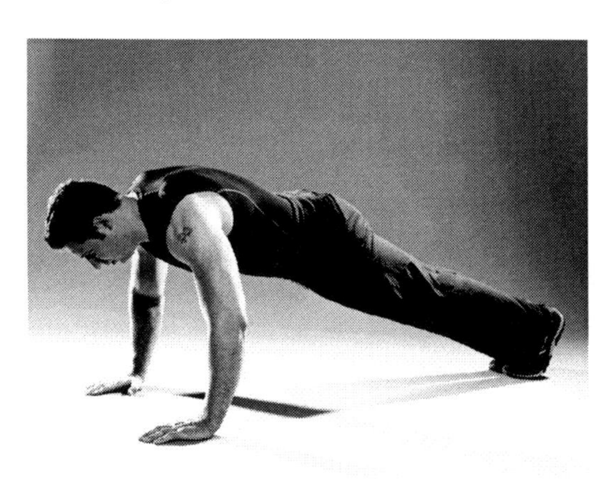

To Perform: Lower yourself in a controlled fashion and pause briefly before raising back up to the starting position. Don't forget to breathe! Do your best to eventually have your nose and/or chest gently touch the floor for optimal range of motion.

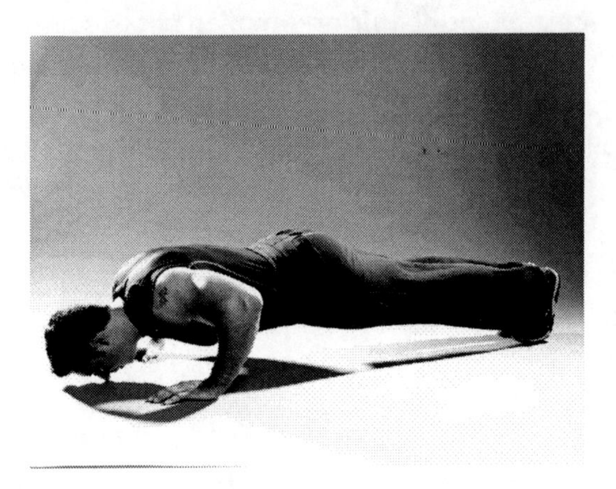

Beginner: Three sets of 10 repetitions
Intermediate: Four sets of 20 repetitions
Advanced: Five sets of 30 repetitions

Rest time between sets should be 30 seconds to two minutes for recovery.

Tips: If this exercise proves to be too difficult, remember to please be patient with your range of motion and be consistent. Be mindful that positioning your feet in a shoulder-width stance would make this exercise easier, but isn't as beneficial for developing the core stabilization muscles. Also, not keeping your feet together would only decrease your progression to perform other push-ups effectively.

3. Staggered Push-ups

This is an advanced exercise since it incorporates more core, shoulder, and triceps stability than the standard Traditional Push-up, and therefore incorporates more strength in your rotator cuffs. This push-up builds lean muscle in the primary movers in this exercise which are: the anterior and medial deltoid muscles, pectoralis major and pectoralis minor muscles, triceps, and gluteus maximus muscles. Moreover, this "staggered" position will aide in creating more overall strength when performing other push-ups that start with your hands shoulder-width apart.

Starting Position: Begin with your arms in a traditional push-up position, then stagger your hands by moving one forward about 6 inches, and the other back about 6 inches, keeping them shoulder-width apart. Your knees, legs, and feet should stay together with your heels up and your body weight forward on your hands, all of which creates a more challenging core workout.

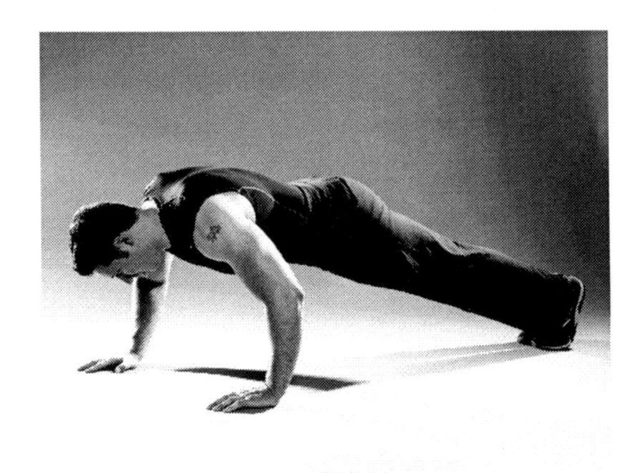

To Perform: Once you rise up from one push-up, execute the next repetition after switching your forward and backward hands. Continue to switch your hand positions between each repetition. The optimal goal is to have your nose and/or chest touch the floor with every "down." Don't forget The Focused Five!

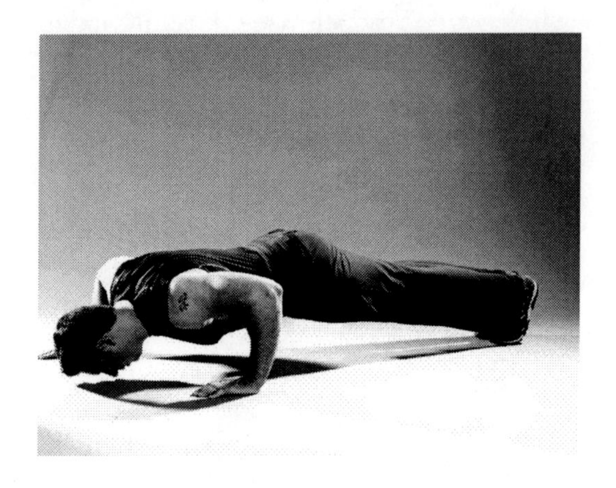

Beginner: Four sets total; two sets each side for 10 repetitions
Intermediate: Six sets total; three sets each side for 16 repetitions
Advanced: Six sets total; three sets each side for 24 repetitions

Rest time between sets should be 30 seconds to three minutes for recovery.

Tips: Particularly when switching the position of your hands between each repetition, it is crucial to maintain a neutral spinal position to engage the core and not hike up your hips. Be mindful not to dip your shoulder or elevate your upper trapezius for strength. If placing your hands staggered six inches proves to be too challenging, you may bring them closer for added stability. However, when that position proves comfortable or easy, challenge yourself by slowing testing just how close to six inches apart you can get them!

4. One-Leg Staggered Push-ups

The first three push-up exercises engaged the core stabilization muscles by keeping the knees, legs, and feet together. After mastering those, this push-up now incorporates the lower body, and therefore challenges the core in a new demanding way by also engaging the core movement muscles such as the erector spinae. This push-up builds lean muscle in the primary movers in this exercise which are: the anterior and medial deltoid muscles, pectoralis major and pectoralis minor muscles, triceps, gluteus maximus muscles, quadriceps, hamstrings, and calves.

Starting Position: Begin with your arms in a traditional push-up position, then stagger your hands by moving one forward about six inches, and the other back about six inches, keeping them shoulder-width apart. Your chest is facing the floor and elbows are only slightly bent. Next, if your right hand is forward in the staggered position, raise your right leg a few inches off the ground while your other foot remains stationary with the heel up. Lock the leg that is in the air at the knee for more hamstring and gluteus maximus muscle recruitment.

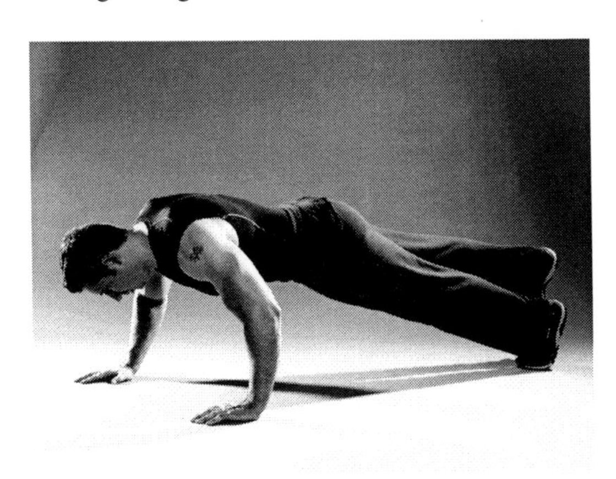

To Perform: Lower your body in a controlled manner while keeping the leg that is in the air stationary throughout. The leg supporting your body should also be locked at the knee throughout. For optimal range of motion, your nose and/or chest should gently touch the floor.

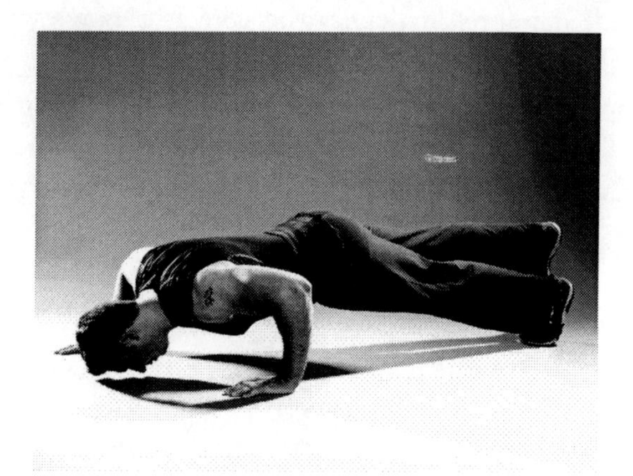

Beginner: Six sets total, two sets each side of 12 repetitions
Intermediate: Six sets total, three sets each side of 16 repetitions
Advanced: Six sets total, three sets each side of 24 repetitions

Rest time between sets should be 30 seconds to three minutes for recovery.

Tips: Be mindful not to raise the leg that is up more than a few inches from the ground. Raising it higher is incorrect form and could result in unnecessary strain to your lower back. Additionally, doing so impedes your ability to maintain a neutral spinal position and therefore does not recruit proper core movement and stabilization muscles. Be mindful to not lean or hike your hips during this push-up, especially while holding one leg up.

5. Alternating Leg Push-ups

This is a challenging power movement that will get more of your lower body involved while building stronger core movement and stabilization muscles in the process. This push-up builds lean muscle in the primary movers of this exercise which are: the anterior and medial deltoid muscles, pectoralis major and pectoralis minor muscles, triceps, gluteus maximus muscles, quadriceps, hamstrings, and calves.

Starting Position: Begin by getting into the Traditional Push-up position with one leg raised about two inches from the floor with your hands placed slightly more than shoulder-width apart.

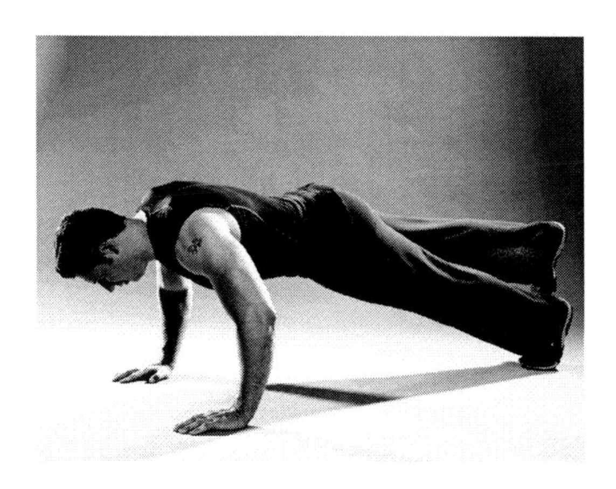

To Perform: With one leg about one to two inches above the floor, lower your body and execute a push-up. The leg that is in the air is locked at the knee to recruit more muscle fibers in your gluteus and hamstring. Before you begin the next repetition, alternate legs with a hop. This "hop" will provide the power in this exercise and should not be more than a few inches from the ground. The optimal goal is to have your nose and/or chest gently touch the floor for optimal range of motion.

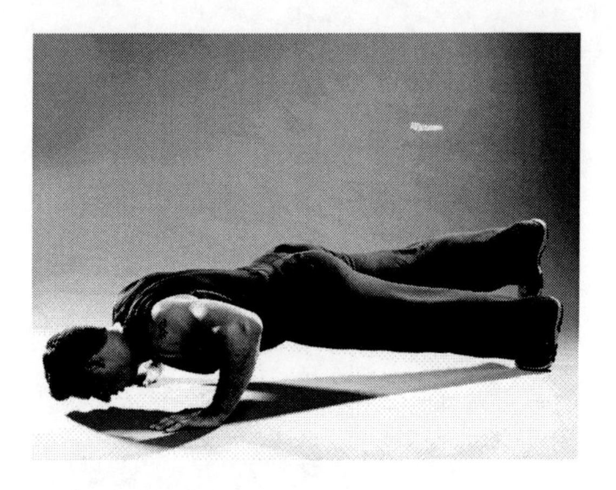

Beginner: Four sets, 15 repetitions each
Intermediate: Five sets, 20 repetitions each
Advanced: Five sets, 30 repetitions each

Rest time between sets should be 30 seconds to three minutes for recovery.

Tips: As stated above, be vigilantly aware of not raising the leg more than a few inches from the ground. Raising it too high can jeopardize the crucial neutral spinal position needed in this exercise for optimal engagement of the core movement and stabilization muscles. Do your best to maintain the power needed for proper execution in this movement by starting the "hopping" motion as you rise up. Remember, as always, not to lean or hike your hips upwards while performing this powerful movement. Lastly, do not drop your shoulder or elevate your upper trapezius. Engage your gluteus maximus muscles, "draw in" your abdominals for strength, and utilize the in/out breaths – all of The Focused Five.

6. Slap Push-ups

At this mid-point of your push-up journey you are beginning to effectively engage your core stabilization and movement muscles and keep your hands stable with movement in your legs. This push-up, if executed correctly, is extremely difficult because it is a functional challenge as much as it is a strength training exercise. Notably, when arm movements are involved in push-ups, the core stabilization and movement muscles must correctly perform the exercise for optimal efficiency. It's easy to perform this push-up with inefficient form. Done efficiently, this exercise will provide a tremendous amount of shoulder, triceps, and rotator cuff stability. It also challenges your hip flexors and psoas muscles since there can be absolutely no leaning to either side. This push-up also creates lean muscle in the primary movers such as: the anterior and medial deltoid muscles, pectoralis major and pectoralis minor muscles, triceps, and gluteus maximus muscles.

Starting position: As in the above techniques, keep your knees, legs, and feet together to engage your core and maintain a neutral spinal position. Next, place your hands slightly more than shoulder-width apart.

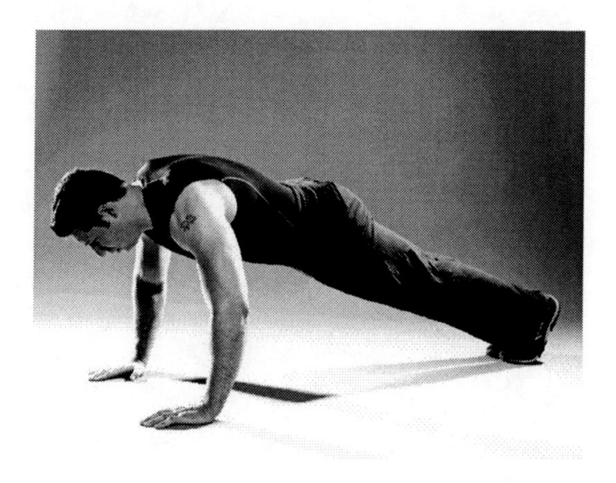

To Perform: Lower into a traditional push-up and as you lift your body up from the ground to return to the starting push-up position, quickly "slap" one hand on your opposite shoulder and return your hand back to the ground to stabilize your body. Next, execute another push-up, lowering your body toward the ground and repeating the slap with the opposite hand at the end/top of the push-up. Develop a consistent tempo or speed when performing these alternating-sides movements. The optimal goal is to have your nose and/or chest touch the floor for optimal range of motion.

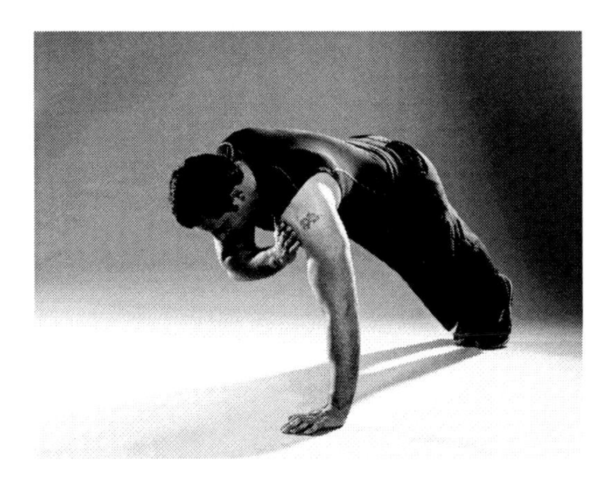

Beginner: Three sets total, 12 repetitions each
Intermediate: Four sets total, 16 repetitions each
Advanced: Four sets total, 24 repetitions each

Rest time between sets should be 30 seconds to three minutes for recovery.

Tips: The trick is not to allow any leaning of your body or any hip hiking in your core. For added strength, "draw in" your abdominals and engage your gluteus maximus muscles. Remember to stay controlled during this exercise, especially when it comes to moving your hands. Place your hands down gently on the ground after each slap. If this exercise proves to be too difficult, position your hands wider than shoulder-width apart. This position will create more stabilization and engage more secondary muscles for support.

7. In to Out Push-ups

This is an advanced exercise for the core stabilization and movement muscles because it incorporates arms movements from side to side with extreme hand placement. This exercise creates a compound amount of shoulder and triceps stability from the first to final repetition due to its hand positioning. This push-up also creates lean muscle in the primary movers such as: the anterior and medial deltoid muscles, pectoralis major and pectoralis minor muscles, triceps, and gluteus maximus muscles. At this point in the push-up journey, your core stabilization and movement muscles are strong, and therefore they will assist the shoulder and triceps with the strength needed for optimal performance.

Starting Position: Position yourself with your chest facing the ground and your hands should be positioned slightly more than shoulder-width apart. Your knees, feet, and legs are together to promote optimal core stability.

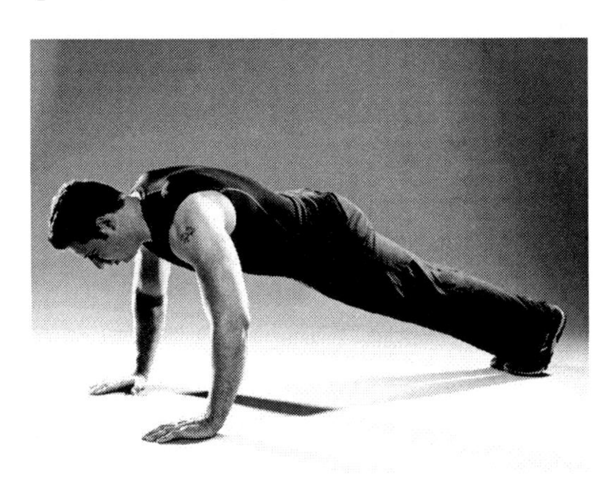

To Perform: Start by executing a push-up with your hands touching one another and rise back up to the starting position. Next, move your hands out continuously a few inches from one another and then perform a push-up. Continue to perform three more push-ups, moving your hands a few more inches apart with every repetition. After performing four repetitions, your hands should be positioned more than shoulder-width apart. To finish a completed round, keep executing push-ups while bringing your hands together a few inches with each repetition until you are back at the starting position with your hands touching. If done correctly, you should execute four push-ups out and then four push-ups in for one full round. As with all push-ups, the paramount goal is to have your nose and/or chest touch the floor for optimal range of motion.

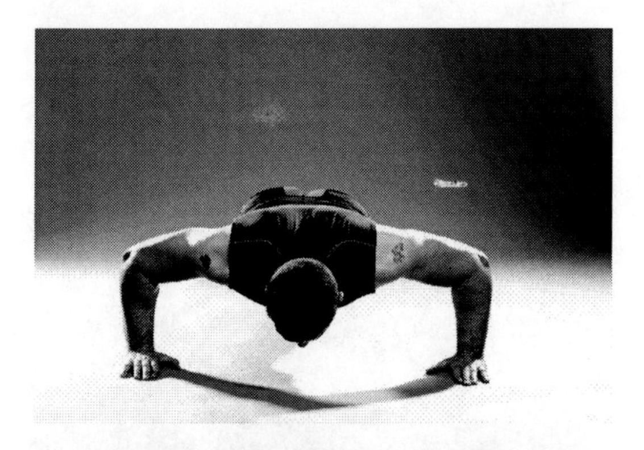

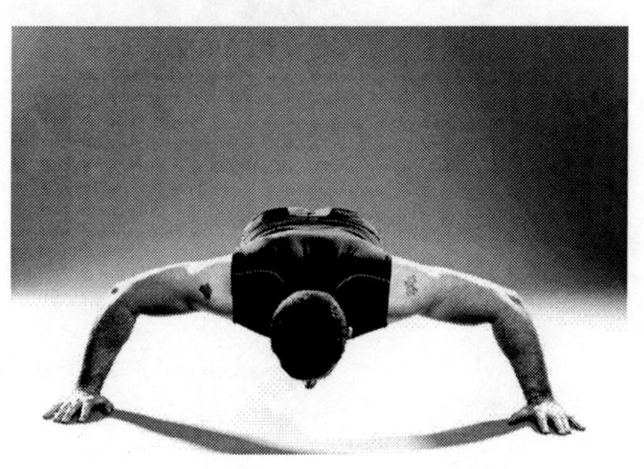

Beginner: Three sets total; one set is considered two rounds of performing four push-ups out and then four push-ups in.
Intermediate: Four sets total; one set is considered three rounds of performing four push-ups out and then four push-ups in.
Advanced: Four sets total; one set is considered five rounds of performing four push-ups out and then four push-ups in.

Rest time between sets should be 30 seconds to three minutes for recovery.

Tips: Be mindful not to move your hands more than a few inches apart while performing each push-up. The core stabilization and movement muscles engage more efficiently with smaller hand placements. Additionally, maintain a neutral spinal position throughout, especially when moving your hands outward past your shoulders. Your gluteus maximus muscles should be engaged throughout for added strength. And don't forget the upward/downward breaths!

8. Staggered Moving Push-ups

This is an advanced exercise for the core stabilization and movement muscles since it incorporates staggered arm movements. Again, push-ups become significantly more challenging when your upper body is in motion. As with any staggered position push-up, this is a beneficial exercise for shoulders, triceps, and for rotator cuff stability. This push-up builds lean muscle in the primary movers in this exercise which are: the anterior and medial deltoid muscles, pectoralis major and pectoralis minor muscles, triceps, and gluteus maximus muscles. Much like the Slap Push-up, this particular exercise challenges the hip flexors and psoas muscles not to lean, creating optimal core efficiency.

Starting Position: Begin with your arms in a traditional push-up position, then stagger your hands by moving one forward about six inches, and the other back about six inches, keeping them slightly more than shoulder-width apart. Your knees, legs, and feet should all be together while your heels are up and rotated slightly forward.

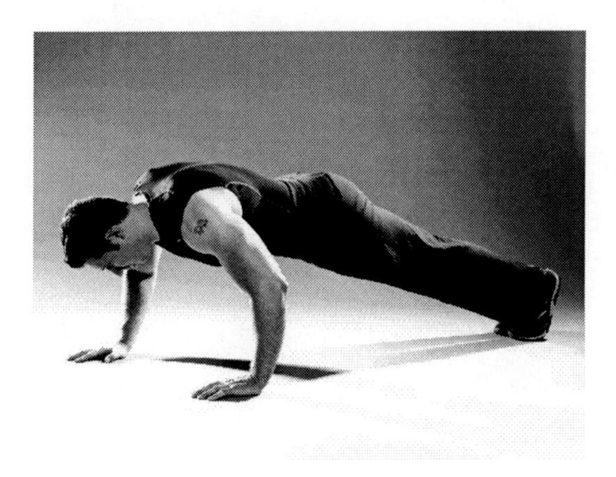

To Perform: From one push-up to the next, switch the hands in a staggered position from one another at the top of the push-up while moving your hands gently from repetition to repetition on the floor. The ultimate goal is to have your nose and/or chest touch the floor for optimal range of motion.

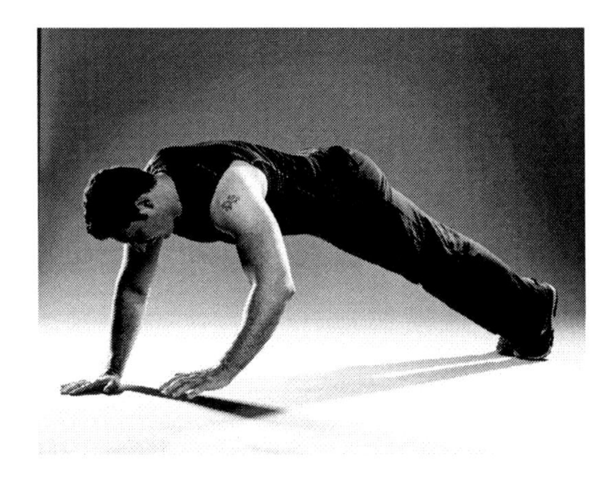

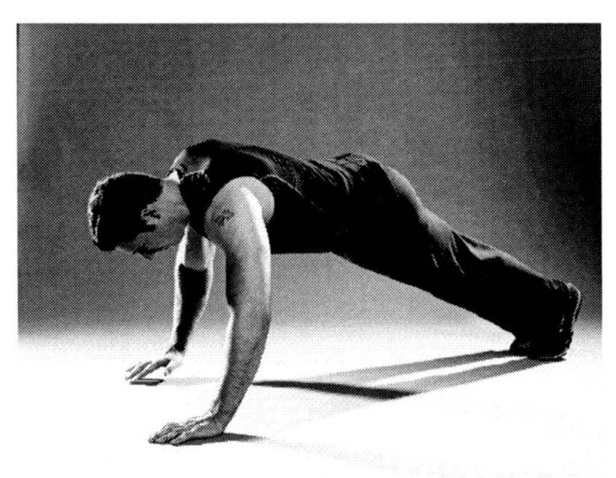

Beginner: Three sets total, 16 repetitions each
Intermediate: Three sets total, 24 repetitions each
Advanced: Four sets total, 30 repetitions each

Rest time between sets should be 30 seconds to three minutes for recovery.

Tips: Remember The Focused Five, particularly keeping your core at a neutral spinal position throughout. Do not lean, shift, or hike your hips during this push-up. Furthermore, be mindful to not dip your shoulders or elevate your upper trapezius for strength. Remember to place your hands down softly on the ground from one repetition to the next. You do not want to place your hands down too forcefully; this could cause potential injury to your wrist or shoulder. If positioning your hands a little more than shoulder-width apart becomes too challenging, you may position your hands wider than the shoulders for added core stability. However, when that position is no longer challenging, attempt the push-up with the previous more challenging position.

9. Walk Out Push-ups

After mastering moving your hands in a staggered position and then moving them side-to-side while keeping your feet stationary in the previous push-ups, the next progression is to move your hands forward and backward. This exercise challenges the core stabilization and movement muscles with optimal effectiveness by adjusting your hand placement to reach far past the shoulder-width position of a traditional push-up. Additionally, the farther you bring your hands forward, the more your hamstrings and calves will become engaged, and therefore stretched in the process. This push-up builds lean muscle in the primary movers in this exercise which are: the anterior and medial deltoid muscles, pectoralis major and pectoralis minor muscles, triceps, gluteus maximus muscles, quadriceps, hamstrings, and calves. At this stage of your push-up journey, your core stabilization and movement muscles are very strong. Thus, they will aide with the shoulder and triceps strength needed for optimal performance.

Starting Position: As with the other push-up beginning stances, keep your knees, legs, and feet together to properly engage your core and maintain a neutral spinal position in your back. Next, place your hands slightly more than shoulder-width apart. The key goal here is to have your nose and/or chest touch the floor for optimal range of motion.

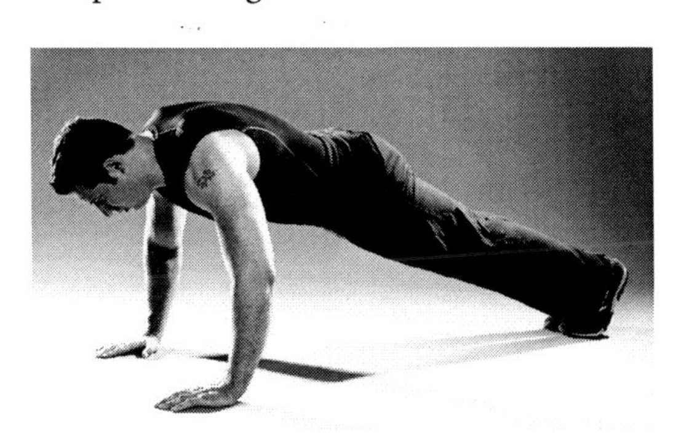

To Perform: Lower yourself until your nose or chest touches the floor and then rise back up to the starting position. Next, move both hands slightly forward a few inches in between each push-up. To finalize a complete round, move or "walk" your hands backwards two inches in between each push-up repetition until they are back at the starting position. For optimal effectiveness, attempt six repetitions forward and then six repetitions backward for one complete round.

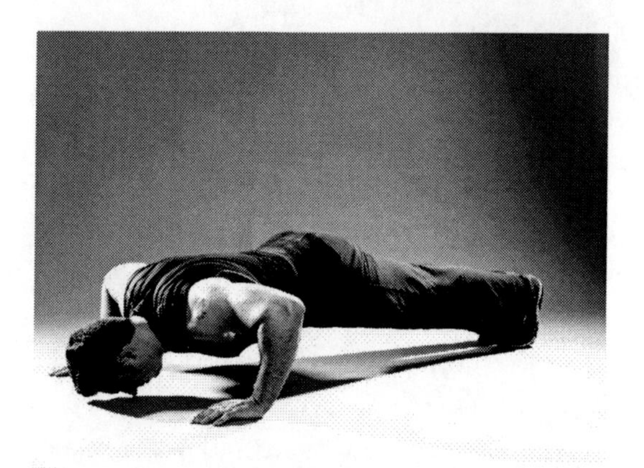

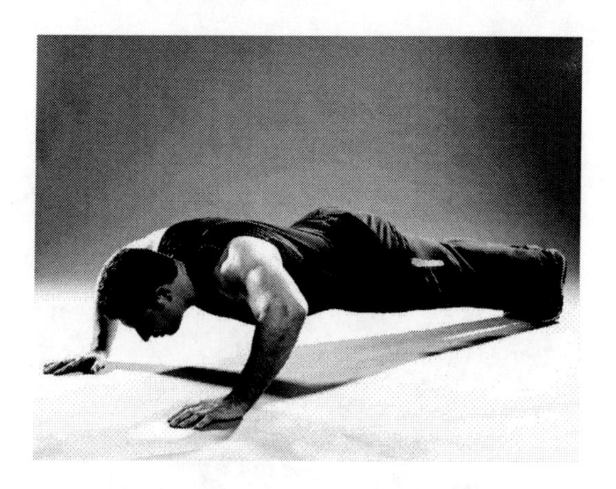

Beginner: Three sets total; one set is considered two rounds of performing six push-ups forward and then six push-ups backward.
Intermediate: Three sets total; one set is considered three rounds of performing six push-ups forward and then six push-ups backward.
Advanced: Four sets total; one set is considered four rounds of performing six push-ups forward and then six push-ups backward.

Rest time between sets should be 30 seconds to three minutes for recovery.

Tips: It's crucial for the core to maintain a neutral spinal position during this movement since your hands are moving forward and then backward continuously. Do not be tempted to move your lower body while performing this push-up. Every muscle below the pelvis must remain stationary for optimal core recruitment. Also, be cautious not to elevate your upper trapezius muscles for strength when bringing your hands forward. Remember to take small steps with your hands for proper core engagement and place your hands softly on the ground with each repetition to not aggravate the shoulders or wrists.

10. Push-ups with Slow-Moving Mountain Climbers

This exercise challenges your lower and upper body for optimal core recruitment due to the duration of time it takes to complete a full set. Foremost, your upper body muscles are completely engaged throughout, both in movement and stabilization, during this push-up. The time under tension that this push-up produces is phenomenal both for function and aesthetic goals. Moreover, the mountain climber portion of this push-up can be considered as "horizontal running." This exercise will also produce lean muscle in your gluteus maximus muscles, hamstrings, quadriceps, and calves. Other primary movers in this exercise are: the anterior and medial deltoid muscles, pectoralis major and pectoralis minor muscles, and triceps.

Starting Position: Begin with your chest facing the ground with your hands slightly more than shoulder-width apart. Your knees, feet, and legs are together to promote optimal core stability.

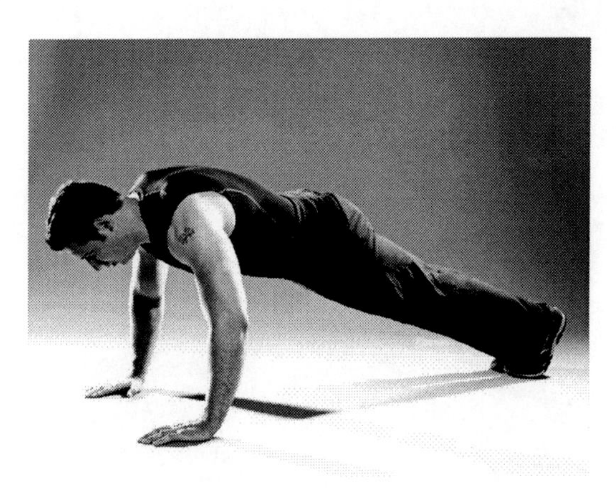

To Perform: Lower yourself into a push-up until your nose or chest gently touches the ground. After completing the push-up, rise up and keep your elbows slightly bent while bending one knee, bringing it to your chest slowly while your other foot remains stationary on the ground with your heel up. Then repeat the same action with your other leg. Performing one push-up and two slow moving mountain climbers with each leg equals one full repetition.

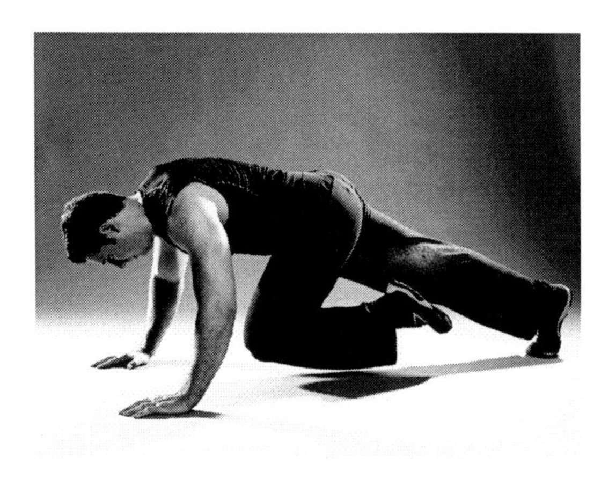

Beginner: Three sets total, 16 repetitions each
Intermediate: Four sets total, 20 repetitions each
Advanced: Four sets total, 30 repetitions each

Rest time between sets should be 30 seconds to three minutes for recovery.

Tips: Remember to always keep your elbows bent to keep tension on the core and upper body muscles. Be especially deliberate when performing the mountain climber portion of this push-up. Traditionally, mountain climbers can be considered a cardiovascular exercise. However, for the time under tension that this exercise provides, they should be done *slowly*. Range of motion is critical too when executing the mountain climber and therefore, your knee should touch the bottom of your chest on each repetition. As always, maintain a neutral spinal position during this push-up and do not be tempted to round your back when attempting to have your knee touch your chest. Don't forget The Focused Five!

11. Push-ups with Reach

Much like the Slap Push-up and Staggered Moving Push-up, this is an even more advanced exercise that challenges the core for optimal efficiency since one arm will be stabilizing your body weight for a longer period of time than during the other push-ups. This exercise creates a tremendous amount of stability in the upper body, and therefore strength in your rotator cuffs, shoulders, and triceps. This push-up, much like the previous two mentioned above, challenges your hip flexors and psoas muscles since there can be absolutely no leaning. This push-up also creates lean muscle in the primary movers such as: the anterior and medial deltoid muscles, pectoralis major and pectoralis minor muscles, triceps, and gluteus maximus muscles.

Starting Position: To begin, start in the traditional push-up position with your knees, feet, and legs together. Your hands should be positioned slightly more than shoulder-width apart.

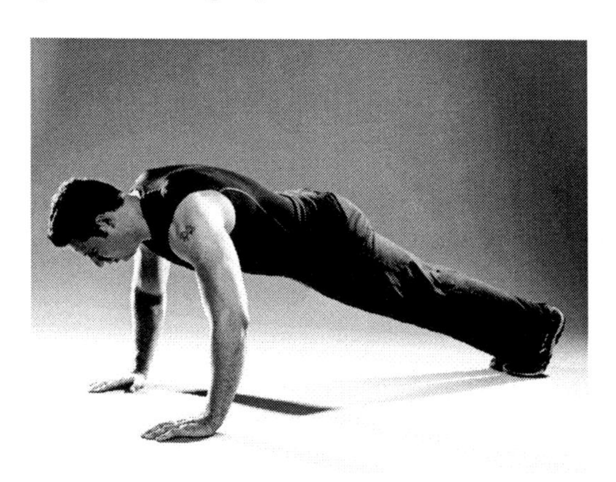

To Perform: Lower into a push-up. Then, as you rise up to the starting position slowly without leaning or hiking your hips, extend and hold one arm fully while locking your elbow at shoulder-level for a full two seconds. Place your hand back on the floor in a controlled fashion and then repeat with your other arm. Performing one push-up and extending both arms outward is one repetition.

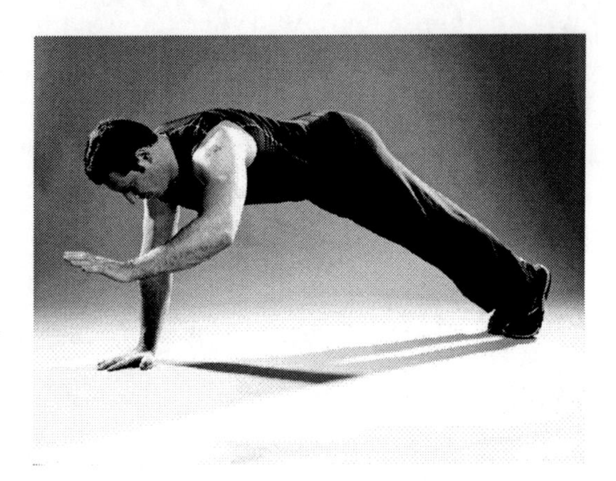

Beginner: Three sets total, eight repetitions with two-second holds
Intermediate: Four sets total, 12 repetitions with two-second holds
Advanced: Four sets total, 16 repetitions with two-second holds

Rest time between sets should be 30 seconds to two minutes for recovery.

Tips: Once more, for absolute core stability there must be little to no movement in your hips. This is incredibly difficult especially on the side which is over-active (tighter) while stabilizing yourself. (To specify: if you are right-dominant, it has traditionally proven to be more challenging when the right hand is on the ground and your left arm is extended.) Thus, continue to bend your elbows and take each repetition slowly to help maintain stability in your hips. Remember also to "draw in" your abdominals, and your gluteus maximus muscles should be engaged throughout for proper strength during this push-up.

12. Crab Walk Push-ups

Your push-up journey is almost complete and every push-up thus far has prepared for you for this last exercise. It contains iswometrics, hand and leg movement, and involves moving your entire body from side to side. Hence, this push-up is the ultimate exercise for creating paramount engagement of the core stabilization and movement muscles. This dynamic movement challenges your muscles intensely to work in an unusual way, creating a high level of coordination while stretching your leg muscles and lower back. Furthermore, this exercise requires cardiovascular ability since your core, upper body, and lower body must work together for optimal strength to aide the hip flexors in maintaining a neutral spinal position throughout. The primary movers in this exercise that build lean muscle are: the anterior, medial, and posterior deltoid muscles; pectoralis major and pectoralis minor muscles; triceps; rhomboids; latissimus dorsi; rotator cuffs; hip flexors; erector spinae; gluteus maximus muscle; hamstrings and calves.

Starting Position: As with most of the push-up beginning positions above, start in the traditional push-up position with your knees, feet, and legs together. Your hands should be positioned slightly more than shoulder-width apart.

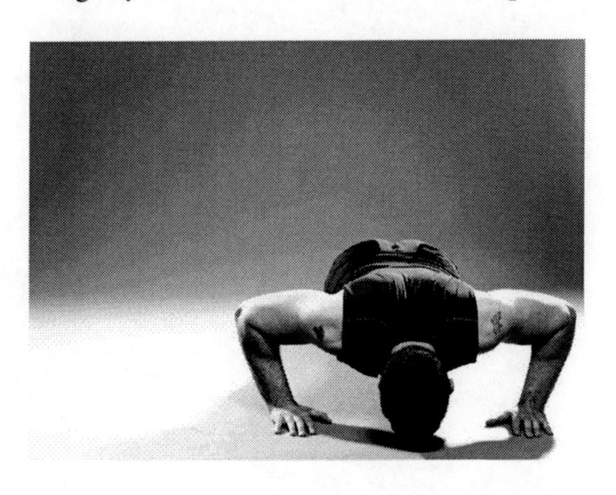

To Perform: Execute a push-up until your nose or chest touches the floor for optimal range of motion, holding for five seconds. Next, rise back up to the starting position and shuffle once sideways with your feet and hands. Your body should end up about one foot from where you started. Continue with another push-up, shuffling back the other direction. To finish a set, alternate from side to side and hold for five seconds for each repetition.

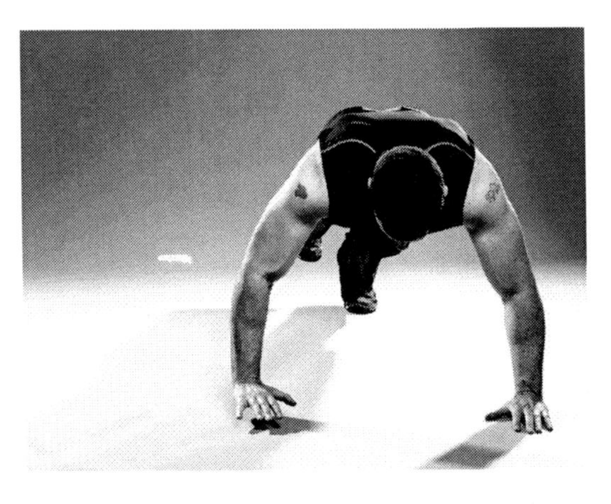

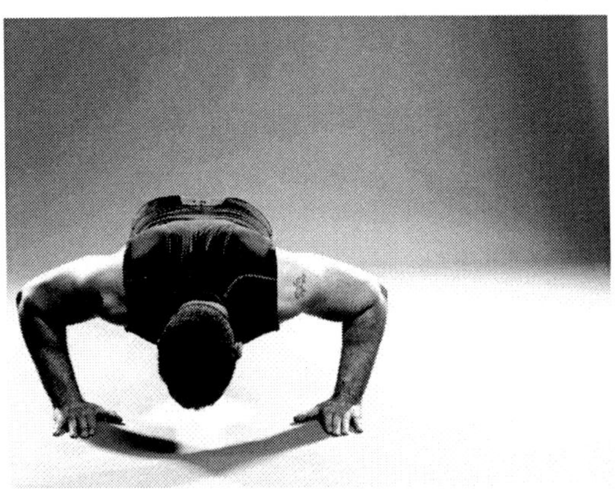

Beginner: Three sets total, 16 repetitions, five-second holds
Intermediate: Four sets total, 20 repetitions, five-second hold
Advanced: Four sets total, 30 repetitions, five-second holds

Rest time between sets should be 30 seconds to two minutes for recovery.

Tips: Remember to maintain a neutral spinal position throughout. Be incredibly cautious not to have your lower back form an inward curve, causing your hips to drop excessively. Similarly, do not round your back, which raises your gluteus maximus muscles higher than your hips. Both of these incorrect methods can cause stress to your lower back without developing functional core strength in the stabilization and movement muscles. If this exercise becomes too strenuous, you may pause and then continue when able. Be mindful to not cross your arms or your feet during this movement, especially if you become fatigued. Crossing will prevent the core from achieving its proper stabilization and movement function, and the rotator cuff will not benefit from optimal stabilization. Finally, challenge yourself to execute these push-ups while applying The Focused Five to their fullest capacity.

Common Muscular Imbalances

Upper Extremity Disorder (UED)– is easy to diagnose since it can best be defined as having protracted shoulders (shoulders that fall forward). The over-active (tight) muscles associated with UED are: the pectoralis major, pectoralis minor, anterior deltoids, and the latissimus dorsi. The muscles that are under-active (weak) are the rhomboids, and the middle and lower trapezius. Those who have UED can still benefit from performing push-ups in order to avoid atrophy in those overactive muscles. However, it is crucial to properly stretch the over-active muscles while strengthening the under-active muscles. For example, execute the wall stretch for 30 seconds to stretch your pectoralis major, pectoralis minor, and anterior deltoids. Applying self-myofacial release by stretching your latissimus dorsi with a foam roller can be extremely effective. Hold the pose for 20 to 30 seconds. Remember to stretch your dominant side one to two more times to encourage symmetry in the body. To strengthen the weak muscles such as the rhomboids, do the pronated dumbbell row. You can stabilize yourself with a weight bench or against the weight rack while you row underneath your chest while holding the dumbbell with your palms down, keeping a slight arch in your back. Perform the row with a weight you can comfortably lift for three sets of eight repetitions. It is important to minimize the effects of UED both to prevent injury and to strive for more aesthetically pleasing posture.

Anterior Pelvic Tilt – is one of the most common muscular imbalances currently in our population. It can best be defined as the pelvis tilting extremely forward. It can be easy to spot in the mirror if you turn sideways when looking at yourself. You do not want to have an excessive arch in your lower back when standing. This arching occurs from a combination of over-active and under-active muscles. The over-active (tight) muscles are the hip flexors (iliacus and psoas muscles) and erector spinae. The under-active (weak) muscles are the gluteus maximus, gluteus medius, and gluteus minimus. You may still perform push-ups with an anterior pelvic tilt; however, it may prove difficult to perform and maintain the neutral spinal position. For that reason, it's critical to strengthen and stretch those specific muscles to prevent your pelvis from tilting forward. For instance, stretch the hip flexor muscles and erector spinae by utilizing a foam roller. The foam roller is a great tool for providing release to these muscles. Hold each stretch for 30 seconds. Again, you will want to stretch your dominant side one to two times more than the other. To strengthen the gluteus muscles, perform three sets of eight repetitions of stationary lunges, step-ups, and floor bridges. By correcting an anterior pelvic tilt, you encourage optimal posture and prevent inefficient movement patterns and potential injury.

Conclusion

Be proud of yourself for picking up and reading this book! If you've made it this far, you've obtained a multitude of knowledge in regards to the core, the push-up, and their benefits. After completing your own push-up journey, you will have acquired more functional core strength, more lean muscle throughout your body, stronger stability in your joints, overall power, and proper posture. Moreover, and most importantly, you will be much healthier! I admire your commitment and dedication to transforming your body by taking this journey with me. Now you can fully appreciate how the push-up can be a tremendous cardiovascular workout along with anaerobically working the upper body, lower body, and core. I realize that many of these push-ups may have been challenging and that this may not have been the easiest of journeys. Remember, though, that not all accomplishments easily change you both physically and mentally. Also bear in mind that no matter your overall fitness performance levels, you can always progress these push-ups further by performing more sets, more repetitions, or by taking shorter rest periods. You may have completed this program, but the journey doesn't have to end. Let this book be the beginning of your own long-term journey, and integrate your favorite – or most challenging – push-ups into your other fitness routines. You now have the foundation of a lifetime of fitness. Let it be your guide to a healthier and stronger you!

I wish you continued success and the best of health throughout this push-up journey and beyond.

About the Author

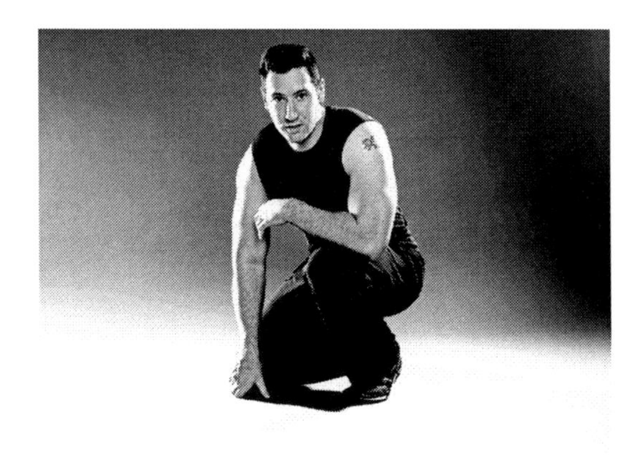

The son of a professional bodybuilder, **Shaun Zetlin** was exposed to weightlifting and exercise at a very young age. After overcoming his own personal physical limitations of being born with clubfeet and deficient gross motor skills, Shaun makes it his mission to share his passion and knowledge of physical fitness and nutrition to help others strive to meet their health goals.

Shaun has successfully run his own personal training business in the New York Metro area for over 10 years, focusing on: strength training, power techniques, corrective injury training, and core stability training. In addition to the highly regarded Master Trainer status, some of his National Academy of Sports Medicine certifications include: Certified Personal Trainer, Pre and Post Natal, Corrective Exercise Practices, Cardiovascular Weight Loss Specialist, Youth Training, and Senior Citizen

Training. Additionally, he is certified by the International Sports Science Association (ISSA) as a Sports Performance Nutrition Specialist.

Shaun earned his Bachelors degree in English Literature and Writing from the University of Delaware. His articles, program designs, and award-winning tips have been published and featured in a variety of books, magazines, and websites including: Price World Publishing, Weight Watchers, Demos Medical Publishing, Brides, Prevention, OnFitness Magazine, Fitness Magazine, and GO: AirTran Magazine.

Shaun also has media experience in both television and radio, ranging from being a fitness model to hosting his own weekly radio fitness show.

For more information about Shaun Zetlin, visit: http://www.zetlinfitness.com/